Knee Pain

Exercises to Increase Flexibility and Stability in Your Knees

(Best Exercises for Knee Arthritis, Mobility, Stiffness, Knee Pain and Rehabilitation)

Christopher Hamilton

Published By **Cathy Nedrow**

Christopher Hamilton

Knee Pain: Exercises to Increase Flexibility and Stability in Your Knees (Best Exercises for Knee Arthritis, Mobility, Stiffness, Knee Pain and Rehabilitation)

ISBN   978-0-9949563-4-7

No part of this guidebook shall be reproduced in any form without permission in writing from the publisher except in the case of brief quotations embodied in critical articles or reviews.

Legal & Disclaimer

Table Of Contents

Chapter 1: Understanding Osteoarthritis In The Knee

What is Osteoarthritis?

The maximum hooked up shape of arthritis is osteoarthritis (OA), a chronic degenerative infection that influences the joints. As a outcome of the gradual loss of cartilage, the cushioning substance that serves as a marvel absorber on the ends of the bones, arthritis is frequently referred to as "placed on and tear" arthritis. The bones of the joint rub in competition to each different as the cartilage deteriorates, ensuing in pain, stiffness, and absence of motion. Any joint in the body can be impacted by means of manner of this tool, regardless of the fact that the hips, knees, arms, and determination are the most customarily affected. Age, trauma, weight troubles, heredity, and osteoarthritis are all causes of the condition. It is seemed as a continual sickness, because of this that it may be handled but now not cured over a prolonged period.

Causes of Osteoarthritis

Although the precise aetiology of osteoarthritis isn't always actually identified, a few variables, which include the following, are belief to be responsible:

Age: As someone ages, their joints wear down and cartilage can also in the end degrade. This will increase the threat of osteoarthritis in aged human beings.

Injury: Osteoarthritis is more liable to broaden in joints that have been broken or subjected to repetitive pressure.

Genetics: Some humans can be predisposed genetically to getting osteoarthritis, which shows that the scenario runs of their own family.

Obesity: Carrying spherical excess weight places greater strain at the joints, particularly the hips and knees, which can also additionally cause osteoarthritis.

Overuse within the place of business or sports activities sports sports: People who paintings in occupations or take part in sports activities that require heavy lifting or repetitive motions are at a better chance of developing osteoarthritis.

Overuse: People who engage in heavy lifting or who are professional athletes may additionally additionally have osteoarthritis due to the use of a joint excessively.

Osteoarthritis chance can also be extended with the aid of manner of other medical illnesses which consist of rheumatoid arthritis, gout, and metabolic issues like hemochromatosis.

It's important to don't forget that distinctive subjects also can in all likelihood make a contribution to it. According to severa studies, hormonal changes, in particular in menopausal ladies, might also moreover make a contribution to the onset of osteoarthritis. Smoking also can improve the chance of getting osteoarthritis and special fitness issues, in step with some research.

It's additionally crucial to preserve in mind that numerous factors might also combine to create osteoarthritis, and the equal person may moreover have high-quality motives for the identical illness. Working with a healthcare specialist permit you to perceive the perfect motives for your osteoarthritis and the simplest control method for the sickness.

A in addition trouble in osteoarthritis is the abnormal joint or bone shape, which may additionally moreover region extra pressure on certain joints and boom their susceptibility to place on and tear. For example, those who are knock-kneed or bowlegged can be extra prone to getting osteoarthritis of their knee joint. Similarly to this, those who've immoderate arches or flat feet may be more vulnerable to getting osteoarthritis of their ankle and foot joints.

Osteoarthritis danger can also be extended by way of manner of many illnesses, which incorporates lupus and rheumatoid arthritis. Osteoarthritis also can furthermore arise because of the contamination those ailments may also additionally produce in the joints, which reasons cartilage to turn out to be worse.

It's additionally essential to have a look at that osteoarthritis is probably exacerbated via terrible diet plan. Deficits in eating regimen D and calcium can also moreover weaken bones, which could decorate the hazard of osteoarthritis with the aid of developing the strain on the joints.

In quit, osteoarthritis is a complicated sickness that can be delivered on thru numerous motives, together with age, trauma, heredity, weight troubles, overuse within the place of job or in a few unspecified time inside the destiny of sports activities, overuse, underlying ailments, and horrible diet plan. To perceive the pleasant reasons for your osteoarthritis and the fantastic course of remedy to manipulate the contamination, it's far critical to appearance a healthcare expert.

Risk Factors

Many threat elements might make a person much more likely to have osteoarthritis. These include:

Age: The hazard of having osteoarthritis rises with advancing years.

Gender: Compared to guys, women have a higher threat of growing osteoarthritis.

Obesity: Carrying spherical extra weight places greater stress on the joints, growing the chance of osteoarthritis.

Joint damage: Osteoarthritis is extra liable to make bigger in joints which have handed via repetitive stress or have been damaged.

Genetics: Some individuals can be predisposed genetically to getting osteoarthritis, which suggests that the scenario runs in their family.

Overuse within the administrative center or sports activities: People who paintings in occupations or participate in sports activities activities that require heavy lifting or repetitive motions are at a better risk of growing osteoarthritis.

Osteoarthritis risk can also be raised via other medical ailments which consist of rheumatoid arthritis, gout, and metabolic problems like hemochromatosis.

Poor nutrients: Vitamin D and calcium deficiency may additionally bring about weakening bones, that could enhance the threat of osteoarthritis and located greater stress on the joints.

abnormal joint or bone shape: Persons who're bowlegged or knock-kneed may be much more likely to get osteoarthritis of their knees, and people who've flat ft or excessive arches may be more likely to build up the situation of their foot and ankle joints.

Symptoms of Osteoarthritis

People may in all likelihood have special osteoarthritis symptoms and signs and symptoms, however, the following are the most everyday ones:

Pain: The maximum ordinary signal of osteoarthritis is pain. Usually, inside the damaged joint, the ache is probably moderate or aching. After exertion or on the same time as the joint is being implemented, it is able to be worse.

Stiffness: Another conventional signal of osteoarthritis is stiffness. Particularly in the morning or after an prolonged length of sitting, the joint may also moreover enjoy tight and difficult to move.

Swelling: The damaged joint may additionally swell, which may additionally make it sense heat to touch.

Reduced variety of motion: As the cartilage inside the joint deteriorates, movement of the joint may also moreover become more difficult. A restricted range of motion would likely give up end result from this.

Bone spurs: Around the joint, tiny bony growths known as bone spurs may moreover shape at the same time because the bones scrape closer to one another.

Crepitus: A cracking or crackling sound or feeling in a joint within the course of movement.

Pain may be added on through difficult motions or sports activities however no longer constantly by way of easy ones.

Additionally, feasible signs and signs embody fatigue, unhappiness, and sleep problems.

It's essential to maintain in thoughts that no longer everybody with osteoarthritis well-known all of these signs and symptoms and signs and symptoms; some human beings may match thru minor symptoms, whilst others can also enjoy intense signs and symptoms and signs. Additionally, it's far essential to get clinical recommendation to have an accurate prognosis and rule out every other trouble that would gift with the identical symptoms.

DIAGNOSIS AND SELF-ASSESSMENT

How to apprehend the signs and symptoms and signs and symptoms and symptoms of Osteoarthritis

There are many signs and signs and signs and symptoms that osteoarthritis may be present. Here are a few techniques for recognizing the signs and signs and symptoms and symptoms and signs and symptoms and signs and symptoms of osteoarthritis:

Joint ache: Pain in the joint is one of the most commonplace symptoms of osteoarthritis. The pain is probably slight or painful, and it is able to grow to be worse after carrying out physical hobby or even as the usage of the affected joint.

Stiffness: Another common symptom of osteoarthritis is stiffness in the afflicted joint, particularly in the morning or after spending pretty a few time sitting down.

Swelling: Osteoarthritis can also be gift if there can be swelling or infection inside the joint.

Reduced sort of motion: As the cartilage in the joint deteriorates, movement of the joint might also moreover grow to be extra difficult. This can also additionally furthermore bring about a restricted variety of movement, every different indication of osteoarthritis.

Bone spurs: Around the joint, tiny bony growths known as bone spurs also can moreover shape while the bones scrape towards one another. These spurs, which might be a symptom of osteoarthritis, may be felt or seen on an x-ray.

Crepitus: When shifting, there can be a popping or crackling sound within the joint. This is a symptom of osteoarthritis.

It's vital to consider that now not all people who has osteoarthritis may additionally need to have all of those signs and symptoms and signs and symptoms; a few human beings can also simplest undergo minor signs and symptoms, on the equal time as others can also additionally enjoy excessive signs and symptoms and signs and symptoms. Osteoarthritis may be efficaciously identified with the help of a healthcare expert, collectively with an orthopaedic medical doctor, rheumatologist, or circle of relatives scientific doctor. To confirm the assessment, they may do a physical examination, report a affected person's scientific records, and request imaging assessments like x-rays or MRIs. Additionally, they might do extra tests like joint aspiration or joint fluid evaluation to look for inflammatory markers.

It's moreover vital to keep in mind that rheumatoid arthritis and gout also can additionally show off signs and symptoms and symptoms which is probably much like the ones of osteoarthritis. Therefore, it's miles important to are seeking out scientific advice to have a accurate assessment and rule out unique sicknesses.

It's critical to document your signs, which includes their occurrence, severity, and demanding or easing elements. Your healthcare company can also locate this data beneficial in identifying the fantastic path of remedy on your osteoarthritis.

Additionally, it's vital to attain this to control your signs and prevent the situation from becoming worse if you have any osteoarthritis signs. Exercise, bodily remedy, weight control, and remedy can also all fall underneath this class. Surgery may be advocated in immoderate situations. It's important to collaborate cautiously collectively with your healthcare company to create a treatment technique that is appropriate for you.

Self-assessment quiz

Here are a few self-assessment quiz questions to see whether or not or now not or now not you will be displaying osteoarthritis signs and symptoms and signs:

Do you've got were given have been given aches or pains in any of your joints?

Do you revel in ache or pain in one or greater of your joints?

Do you have stiffness in your joints, especially in the morning or after sitting for an extended length?

Do you have got got trouble transferring one or extra of your joints?

Do you've got swelling or infection in one or greater of your joints?

Have you observed any adjustments on your joint like deformity, crepitus (cracking or popping sound or sensation within the joint while moving) or bone spurs?

Does your joint ache or pain make it tough a first-rate manner to carry out each day sports?

Does your joint pain or ache worsen with positive sorts of climate or after exceptional sports activities?

Have you observed any modifications to your usual outstanding of existence because of your joint ache or pain?

If you answered sure to any of those questions, it may be a signal which you are experiencing symptoms of osteoarthritis. It is crucial to are looking for advice from a healthcare expert to get a right analysis and to rule out other conditions.

This self-assessment take a look at might not have addressed all the symptoms and signs and symptoms and symptoms and signs and symptoms and symptoms of osteoarthritis. Furthermore, it's miles critical to go through in mind that the ones queries do no longer serve rather for a certified medical diagnostic. It's essential to look a medical doctor for an correct diagnosis and to rule out precise ailments in case you are displaying any symptoms that fear you.

It's additionally vital to maintain in thoughts that specific people can be stricken by osteoarthritis in severa techniques and that the signs and symptoms may also moreover trade. It's essential to speak with a scientific professional to decide the splendid course of motion on your unique state of affairs.

Chapter 2: Treatment Options Physical Therapy

Physical therapy is crucial for treating osteoarthritis ache and improving joint usual performance. A bodily therapist can also collaborate with you to create a custom designed schooling regimen that takes below interest your precise necessities and goals.

Exercises that growth flexibility, power, and staying strength are regularly part of osteoarthritis bodily treatment. Exercise might also growth cardiovascular health, joint mobility, and muscular help surrounding the joint through range-of-motion, strengthening, and cardio sports.

To deal with pain and inflammation, bodily remedy also can use techniques along side ultrasound, electric powered stimulation, and warmth or cold remedy.

Your bodily therapist can also teach you on how to utilize braces or canes as assistive aids to lessen the stress at the injured joint. They may also moreover display you the way to go approximately your regular commercial enterprise business enterprise in a manner that spares your joint ache.

People with osteoarthritis may additionally benefit from physical remedy with the useful resource of getting better joint feature, lots much less pain, and common higher first-class of lifestyles. It's important to collaborate carefully with a physical therapist to create a treatment method that is suitable in your necessities and desires.

It's also critical to take a look at that, if crucial, surgical treatment need to be combined with bodily treatment in addition to unique remedy alternatives which consist of treatment and weight loss applications. For the quality outcomes, a bodily therapist also can collaborate with exceptional medical examiners which includes rheumatologists, orthopaedic surgeons, and number one care medical docs.

The signs and symptoms and symptoms of osteoarthritis may be controlled with some of bodily remedy strategies. The most commonplace physical treatment strategies for treating osteoarthritis embody the following:

Range-of-movement wearing events: By allowing the joint to transport via its whole style of movement, the ones sporting sports motive to increase joint flexibility and mobility. This might also useful resource in easing stiffness and enhancing joint functionality in desired.

Strengthening wearing sports: Exercises that boom muscular strength and persistence across the injured joint are known as strengthening bodily activities. The threat of damage may be reduced and joint stability may be improved.

Aerobic bodily video games: Workouts that increase cardiovascular fitness and all-spherical bodily function are referred to as aerobic sporting sports. Aerobic carrying sports also can help to reduce pain, enhance joint mobility, and decorate the overall exceptional of lifestyles.

Manual therapy: Physical therapists rent manual remedy, which includes joint manipulation and mobilization, to growth joint mobility and decrease ache and infection.

Cryotherapy and thermotherapy: cryotherapy and thermotherapy. While thermotherapy employs warmth treatment to beautify blood go with the flow and reduce muscular spasms, cryotherapy makes use of cold treatment to alleviate infection.

Electrical stimulation: Physical therapists can also lease electric powered stimulation to useful resource recovery within the injured joint and to reduce ache and infection.

Tape and bracing: To provide more help and stability to the injured joint, bodily therapists can also additionally additionally rent taping or bracing.

Balance and gait schooling: Physical therapists may go with sufferers to beautify balance and gait (on foot fashion) to decrease the danger of falls and boom mobility in large.

Patient education: Physical therapists can also furthermore educate sufferers on the way to use assistive gadgets like canes or walkers efficaciously in addition to a manner to pass about their ordinary lives in a manner that does not vicinity undue stress on the injured joint. Additionally, they will offer schooling on wholesome residing, suitable body mechanics, and damage avoidance.

Self-manipulate: To assist patients in higher controlling their signs and symptoms and signs and symptoms and signs and enhancing joint feature, bodily therapists also can train them self-management techniques which includes at-home stretching and strengthening sports.

It is crucial to preserve in thoughts that the satisfactory bodily treatment strategies hired will rely upon the affected man or woman as someone with their necessities and objectives. A physical therapist will collaborate with the affected person to create a custom treatment plan that takes into consideration all in their necessities and objectives. When crucial, surgical treatment must be mixed with physical remedy further to different remedy alternatives consisting of treatment and weight manage.

MEDICATIONS

To cope with the signs and signs and symptoms of osteoarthritis, a number of pills are available. These embody:

Pain relievers: Nonsteroidal anti-inflammatory drug treatments (NSAIDs), together with ibuprofen (Advil, Motrin), naproxen (Aleve), and acetaminophen (Tylenol), are beneficial in reducing pain and contamination related to osteoarthritis.

Topical analgesics: Localized ache consolation may be finished via utilizing topical analgesics, along aspect creams or gels containing NSAIDs, right away to the pores and pores and pores and skin over the afflicted joint.

Counterirritants: These are menthol or capsaicin-containing lotions, gels, or ointments that may be used to appease pain and enhance joint feature.

Prescription Drugs: If over the counter drug remedies do not paintings, your health practitioner ought to signify stronger pain relievers like tramadol or more potent NSAIDs like celecoxib (Celebrex).

Steroids: Steroids can be used to reduce joint pain and infection. They can be ingested or proper now injected into the joint.

Disease-editing osteoarthritis pills (DMOADs): Many medicinal drugs have been created to lessen the severity of osteoarthritis. These are called DMOADs, and glucosamine, chondroitin sulfate, and hyaluronic acid are some examples.

It's vital to recall that treatment need to be used with unique remedy options which incorporates bodily treatment, weight reduction, and dietary modifications. Although they'll now not resolve the underlying difficulty, drug remedies might alleviate signs and symptoms at the same time as moreover having potentially detrimental effects. It is critical to speak with a clinical expert to determine the great path of movement to your specific situation.

SURGERY

If lots much less invasive restoration approaches like bodily remedy, remedy, and weight reduction have no longer sufficiently relieved osteoarthritis signs and symptoms, surgical remedy can be explored as a therapeutic possibility.

The particular joint concerned and the degree of osteoarthritis will determine the form of surgery this is finished.

Joint opportunity: A surgical gadget referred to as arthroplasty, typically referred to as joint alternative, involves eliminating the diseased joint and replacing it with a prosthetic joint. The knee, hip, and shoulder are the most usually treated joints with this remedy.

Osteotomy: Osteotomy is a surgical treatment wherein the bone is sliced to realign the joint and rebalance the weight-bearing strain. The knee is wherein this remedy is most often finished.

Arthroscopy: Arthroscopy is a minimally invasive surgical remedy that includes putting a tiny digital virtual camera via a small incision into the joint. This remedy may be used to eliminate free pieces of bone or cartilage and to restore tendons or ligaments which have been injured.

Debridement: a surgery that would help to reduce soreness and beautify joint function via casting off the diseased cartilage and bone from the joint.

It's crucial to do not forget that surgical remedy isn't always normally the top notch direction of motion and want to handiest be taken into consideration as a ultimate lodge. Before selecting to have surgical treatment, it's far crucial to thoroughly don't forget the possible benefits and dangers. Surgery includes risks. Before creating a preference, it's also vital to consider the prolonged-term effects due to the fact surgical remedy might not be capable of truly restore joint function. The most suitable route of remedy for each affected individual may be determined with the help of a collection of health workers, along side orthopaedic surgeons, physical therapists, and number one care doctors.

ASSISTIVE DEVICES

Assistive gadgets may be used to assist manipulate osteoarthritis signs and symptoms and signs and symptoms and beautify joint characteristic. These technology may additionally resource with mobility, ache remedy, and standard super of lifestyles.

Canes: Canes are hand-held strolling aids that deliver assist and stability. They may be used to assist shift weight a protracted manner from the joint and alleviate pain.

Walkers: Walkers, like canes, deliver more assist and balance. They may be used by individuals who aren't capable of comply with a cane or who need greater help even as on foot.

Crutches: are transportable devices used to offer help and balance while taking walks. They can be used to assist shift weight faraway from the joint and alleviate pain.

Knee braces: Knee braces can also furthermore assist to help and stabilize the knee joint. They can be implemented to useful resource with pain comfort, joint feature, and damage prevention.

Orthotics: these are gadgets that can be worn in footwear to help shift weight and relieve strain on an injured joint.

These may be created to order or offered off the shelf.

Ramps and handrails: Ramps and handrails may additionally help people with osteoarthritis in navigating stairs and choppy terrain. They may also additionally help in decreasing the danger of falls and enhancing mobility.

It's vital to keep in thoughts that assistive gadgets want to be implemented in mixture with specific healing approaches which consist of physical remedy, remedy, and weight manage. A healthcare professional, collectively with a physical therapist, might also moreover useful resource in identifying the most appropriate assistive device for each particular affected person.

EXERCISE

Exercise is an critical detail in controlling osteoarthritis signs and signs and symptoms. Exercise frequently may additionally moreover assist lower ache, enhance joint feature, and improve the general extraordinary of existence. The kinds of exercise counseled for people with osteoarthritis also can furthermore range relying on the joint and the severity of the osteoarthritis.

Range of motion carrying activities: These physical sports are purported to boom joint flexibility and mobility. These bodily video video games may be used to enhance mobility and decrease stiffness in the afflicted joint.

Strengthening sports activities sports: are intended to assist increase muscular energy whilst also supporting the damaged joint. These wearing sports activities can also additionally assist enhance the stableness of the joint and decrease the threat of falling.

Aerobic physical activities: such as walking, cycling, or swimming, intention to growth cardiovascular health and huge health. These sports activities sports can also moreover assist relieve pain and beautify joint function.

Balance wearing activities: are supposed to help you enhance your balance and stability. These wearing sports can also help lower the threat of falling and beautify modern-day joint feature.

Yoga and tai chi: are low-effect wearing sports which could help increase joint flexibility and mobility, further to decrease pressure and enhance balance.

Before beginning any fitness software program software, it's miles critical to touch a healthcare expert on the side of a physical therapist. They may additionally assist in figuring out the maximum remarkable fitness utility for each affected character and in growing a customized exercising plan.

It is crucial, to start with, low-impact sports activities and little by little increase the depth and duration of the sports because the joint strengthens. It is also essential to keep away from workout exercises that produce pain or discomfort, as well as to prevent exercise if pain arises.

NUTRITION AND DIET

Diet and vitamins are key in controlling osteoarthritis symptoms. Maintaining a wholesome food plan and weight may additionally additionally additionally assist to reduce the strain at the afflicted joint and enhance everyday joint characteristic.

Maintaining a wholesome weight: Excess weight locations greater stress on weight-bearing joints such as the hips, knees, and determination. Weight loss may also moreover assist to lessen the strain on the joint and beautify joint feature.

Consuming anti-inflammatory food: Eating anti-inflammatory ingredients such as cease stop end result, veggies, fish, nuts, and seeds may additionally help to lower contamination inside the body and enhance joint health.

Protein intake: Protein intake is critical for keeping muscle businesses and helping the joint. Fish, chicken, lean meats, and legumes are excessive in protein.

Getting adequate nutrients D and calcium: Vitamins D and calcium are essential for bone health. Fatty fish, egg yolks, and fortified food are rich property of nutrition D, even as dairy merchandise, leafy veggies, and fortified meals are suitable resources of calcium.

Avoiding inflammatory materials: Certain meals, collectively with processed meals, fried substances, and diffused sweets, also can moreover purpose irritation inside the body. These ingredients ought to be averted to assist decrease contamination and decorate joint health.

To growth a tailored nutrients plan, talk with a healthcare professional inclusive of a nutritionist. Based on their desires and health troubles, they may help in identifying the proper weight loss plan and vitamins plan for each affected man or woman.

FOODS TO CONSUME

Fruits and greens: rich in antioxidants and anti inflammatory substances which encompass berries, cherries, pineapple, ginger, turmeric, and leafy greens consisting of spinach, kale, and broccoli.

Fish: Fish robust in omega-three fatty acids, along with salmon, tuna, and sardines, may additionally beneficial resource to lower contamination and decorate joint health.

Nuts and seeds: Anti-inflammatory chemical compounds and accurate fats are ample in nuts and seeds including almonds, walnuts, flaxseed, and chia seeds.

Legumes: Beans, lentils, and peas are wealthy in protein and fibre and can be a outstanding deliver of vitamins for vegetarians and vegans.

Whole grains: which consist of quinoa, brown rice, and oats, are ample in fibre, vitamins, and minerals, and might useful aid in infection discount.

FOODS TO AVOID

Processed meals: along with fast food, snack factors, and prepared-to-eat food, are often wealthy in dangerous fat, carbohydrates, and salt, which can also additionally purpose inflammation and reason weight gain.

Fried food: Fried food are wealthy in dangerous fat and may result in infection. Examples include French fries and fried bird.

Refined sugars: Sugars that have been delicate, together with those found in sweet, cookies, and soda, also can result in inflammation and weight advantage.

Red meat: Saturated fats in beef, together with pork, hog, and lamb, might probably bring about infection.

Alcohol: Excessive alcohol ingesting may also additionally motive infection, weight gain, and different fitness problems.

It's vital to preserve in mind that everyone's nutritional needs range, and contacting a healthcare professional, at the side of a nutritionist, is usually recommended earlier than making any dramatic nutritional adjustments.

30 DAYS MEAL PLAN SAMPLE

Here is an example 30-day meal plan for osteoarthritis control with food and nutrients:

Week 1:

Monday: Breakfast - Oatmeal with blueberries and a sprinkle of flaxseed. Lunch - Grilled salmon with quinoa and steamed broccoli. Dinner - Lentil soup with a facet salad of combined vegetables.

Tuesday: Breakfast - Scrambled eggs with spinach and tomatoes. Lunch -

Turkey and avocado wrap with a thing of candy potato fries. Dinner - Baked chook with brown rice and inexperienced beans.

Wednesday: Breakfast - Greek yoghurt with mixed berries and honey. Lunch - Tuna salad sandwich with a element of fruit. Dinner - Grilled shrimp with cauliflower rice and asparagus.

Thursday: Breakfast - Smoothie bowl with spinach, banana, and almond milk. Lunch - Black bean and vegetable stir-fry with brown rice. Dinner - Stuffed bell peppers with quinoa and floor turkey.

Friday: Breakfast - Whole wheat toast with peanut butter and banana. Lunch - Grilled chicken with a element of roasted sweet potatoes. Dinner -

Vegetable and lentil curry with a element of brown rice.

Saturday: Breakfast - Scrambled eggs with diced onions and bell peppers. Lunch - Turkey and cheese wrap with a aspect of fruit. Dinner - Baked salmon with a facet of quinoa and steamed broccoli.

Sunday: Breakfast - Oatmeal with combined berries and a sprinkle of chia seeds. Lunch - Grilled bird with a facet of roasted veggies. Dinner - Lentil and vegetable soup with a side of blended veggies.

Week 2:

Monday: Breakfast - Greek yoghurt with combined berries and honey. Lunch - Tuna salad sandwich with a detail of fruit. Dinner - Grilled shrimp with cauliflower rice and asparagus.

Tuesday: Breakfast - Smoothie bowl with spinach, banana, and almond milk. Lunch - Black bean and vegetable stir-fry with brown rice. Dinner - Stuffed bell peppers with quinoa and floor turkey.

Wednesday: Breakfast - Whole wheat toast with peanut butter and banana. Lunch - Grilled chicken with a component of roasted candy potatoes. Dinner - Vegetable and lentil curry with a aspect of brown rice.

Thursday: Breakfast - Scrambled eggs with diced onions and bell peppers. Lunch - Turkey and cheese wrap with a aspect of fruit. Dinner - Baked salmon with a side of quinoa and steamed broccoli.

Friday: Breakfast - Oatmeal with blended berries and a sprinkle of chia seeds. Lunch - Grilled fowl with a factor of roasted greens. Dinner - Lentil and vegetable soup with a aspect of combined veggies.

Saturday: Breakfast - Greek yoghurt with mixed berries and honey. Lunch - Tuna salad sandwich with a side of fruit. Dinner - Grilled shrimp with cauliflower rice and asparagus.

Sunday: Breakfast - Smoothie bowl with spinach, banana, and almond milk. Lunch - Black bean and vegetable stir-fry with brown rice. Dinner - Stuffed bell peppers with quinoa and ground turkey.

Week three:

Monday: Breakfast - Whole wheat toast with peanut butter and banana. Lunch - Grilled chicken with a factor of roasted sweet potatoes. Dinner - Vegetable and lentil curry with a facet of brown rice.

Tuesday: Breakfast - Scrambled eggs with diced onions and bell peppers. Lunch - Turkey and cheese wrap with a aspect of fruit. Dinner - Baked salmon with a issue of quinoa and steamed broccoli.

Wednesday: Breakfast - Oatmeal with combined berries and a sprinkle of chia seeds. Lunch - Grilled hen with a aspect of roasted veggies. Dinner - Lentil and vegetable soup with a problem of mixed veggies.

Thursday: Breakfast - Greek yoghurt with blended berries and honey. Lunch - Tuna salad sandwich with a element of fruit. Dinner - Grilled shrimp with cauliflower rice and asparagus.

Friday: Breakfast - Smoothie bowl with spinach, banana, and almond milk. Lunch - Black bean and vegetable stir-fry with brown rice. Dinner - Stuffed bell peppers with quinoa and ground turkey.

Saturday: Breakfast - Whole wheat toast with peanut butter and banana. Lunch - Grilled chook with a side of roasted sweet potatoes. Dinner - Vegetable and lentil curry with a facet of brown rice.

Sunday: Breakfast - Scrambled eggs with diced onions and bell peppers. Lunch - Turkey and cheese wrap with a component of fruit. Dinner - Baked salmon with a thing of quinoa and steamed broccoli.

Week 4:

Monday: Breakfast - Oatmeal with combined berries and a sprinkle of chia seeds. Lunch - Grilled chook with a aspect of roasted vegetables. Dinner - Lentil and vegetable soup with a issue of blended greens.

Tuesday: Breakfast - Greek yoghurt with combined berries and honey. Lunch - Tuna salad sandwich with a aspect of fruit. Dinner - Grilled shrimp with cauliflower rice and asparagus.

Wednesday: Breakfast - Smoothie bowl with spinach, banana, and almond milk. Lunch - Black bean and vegetable stir-fry with brown rice. Dinner - Stuffed bell peppers with quinoa and floor turkey.

Thursday: Breakfast - Whole wheat toast with peanut butter and banana. Lunch - Grilled fowl with a side of roasted sweet potatoes. Dinner - Vegetable and lentil curry with a element of brown rice.

Friday: Breakfast - Scrambled eggs with diced onions and bell peppers. Lunch - Turkey and cheese wrap with a side of fruit. Dinner - Baked salmon with a facet of quinoa and steamed broccoli.

Saturday: Breakfast - Oatmeal with mixed berries and a sprinkle of chia seeds. Lunch - Grilled bird with a issue of roasted veggies. Dinner - Lentil and vegetable soup with a aspect of blended vegetables.

Sunday: Breakfast - Greek yoghurt with blended berries and honey. Lunch - Tuna salad sandwich with a difficulty of fruit. Dinner - Grilled shrimp with cauliflower rice and asparagus.

It is important to do not forget that this meal plan is just an instance and want to be customized to your particular dietary necessities and tastes. Before making any awesome changes on your food regimen, you have to moreover touch a healthcare expert and/or a knowledgeable dietitian.

Chapter 3: Prevention And Management
Tips for Managing Pain

Keep moving: Gentle exercise might probably assist lessen knee ache and stiffness. Walking, swimming, and cycling are excellent low-effect carrying events.

Apply warmth or bloodless remedy to the knee: Applying warmth or bloodless therapy to the knee would probable help relieve pain. An ice % can also moreover help relieve contamination, even as a heating pad or heat bath can offer comforting warmth.

Use assistive gadgets: Using canes, crutches, or knee braces can help relieve stress at the stricken knee and boom mobility.

Try the following over-the-counter ache relievers: Nonsteroidal anti inflammatory drug remedies (NSAIDs) like ibuprofen or naproxen may additionally moreover useful aid with ache remedy and irritation cut price.

Consider dietary supplements: Glucosamine and chondroitin dietary supplements may moreover useful aid with ache consolation and joint health.

Maintain a wholesome weight: Because being obese puts more pressure at the knee, retaining a healthful weight can also additionally help restrict ache and improve popular fitness.

Maintain appropriate posture: Good posture also can assist reduce pressure at the knee and relieve ache.

Try rest strategies: Because stress may worsen ache, relaxation practices like yoga, meditation, or deep respiratory can help decrease anxiety and decorate popular well-being.

Seek medical remedy: If self-discipline strategies are ineffective, it's miles critical to are searching for scientific hobby, considering that there are numerous recovery options to be had.

It's critical to recollect that everybody's ache manipulate necessities range, so it is best to speak with a healthcare professional to find out the extremely good pain management approach for you.

MAINTAINING AN ACTIVE LIFESTYLE

Maintaining an lively life-style is critical for controlling knee osteoarthritis ache. Low-impact physical sports activities like taking walks, swimming, and cycling can also additionally help alleviate knee discomfort and stiffness.

Walking: is a exquisite low-impact interest that could assist improve mobility and decrease knee ache. Begin with small walks and step by step growth the distance as your knee strengthens.

Swimming: is a excellent technique to exercising the knee without setting an excessive amount of strain on it. Water buoyancy relieves strain at the knee, bearing in mind low-effect education.

Cycling: is every different low-impact exercising that would help construct knee strength and alleviate ache. Recumbent motorcycles are an outstanding opportunity for ladies and men stricken by knee pain for the reason that they lessen stress on the knee.

Yoga and stretching: Yoga and stretching can also boom knee flexibility and form of movement. Working with a yoga instructor who can adjust practices in your scenario is ideal.

Strengthening sports activities sports: together with the leg press, leg extension, and leg curl, may also additionally help beautify knee strength and alleviating pain.

Consult a bodily therapist: A physical therapist also can layout a custom designed schooling software program appropriate in your unique requirements, in addition to offer commands at the manner to execute carrying activities effectively to save you destiny damage.

Fitness ought to be completed cautiously, and it is maximum brilliant to touch a healthcare professional in advance than beginning any new exercise regular.

PREVENTIVE MEASURES

Preventive interventions can also help decrease the threat of having osteoarthritis in the knee or halt its course.

Maintain a healthful weight: Because being overweight or obese places extra pressure at the knee, retaining a healthful weight can also help lower the hazard of growing osteoarthritis.

Exercise frequently: Regular exercise may additionally moreover moreover assist improve knee strength and versatility, lowering the threat of growing osteoarthritis.

Wear proper shoes: Wearing shoes with sufficient arch assist and cushioning might also help restriction pressure on the knee and the risk of developing osteoarthritis.

Avoid immoderate-effect sports activities activities: Because high-impact sports like going for walks or leaping region more strain on the knee, warding off them can also furthermore help restriction the hazard of developing osteoarthritis.

Warm the knee: Warming the knee may also additionally help alleviate stiffness and pain. When the knee is cold, use a knee brace or a heating pad to keep it warmness.

Use assistive gadgets: Using canes, crutches, or knee braces can assist relieve strain on the knee and growth mobility.

Get accurate enough calcium and vitamins D: Calcium and nutrition D are critical for wholesome bones, which may additionally assist reduce the hazard of developing osteoarthritis.

Avoid smoking and ingesting carefully: Smoking and excessive alcohol consumption could in all likelihood beautify the hazard of having osteoarthritis.

Remember that everyone's danger elements and necessities are specific, so communicate with a healthcare expert to determine the fantastic preventative actions for you.

Chapter 4: 26 Diy Sore Knee Pain Treatments

You Can Easily Do at Home

Why need to you deal with your knees, rather than someone else? Well, to begin with, we empower ourselves whilst we take responsibility for our non-public nicely being. The truth is, nobody knows better than ourselves what goes on with our our bodies 2nd with the aid of 2nd and minute via minute than we do. Did you apprehend that there are at the least 26 DIY procedures to cope with your knees at home?

By cultivating mindfulness, we are in a much higher function to make modifications and changes. So those 26 Knee Health Secrets can help you get as a minimum brief consolation if you have a massive hassle, and likely a solution for knee ache that you can do yourself.

At this 2d, what feature are you sitting in, slouching or sitting up right away Or perhaps mendacity down. A few nights inside the beyond, I wakened inside the nighttime with my left knee aching. It changed into in a humorous half of twisted position. That's an example.

What's the weather like? Has it modified nowadays and you are noticing pain to your joints?

Another manner too common example of self care is ingesting. Mindless consuming results in weight advantage which results in greater pressure to your joints.

Fact is, overweight people are more likely to have knee problems than those of ordinary weight. Eating healthful elements carefully is step one to better health. Another instance is sports sports. They generally say, "No ache— no advantage", but, such heroics can bring about strains or long term harm. Knowing the distinction between strong ache and volatile pain is the important factor detail.

"I ought to Treat Pain in My Knees … But How?"

Getting proper right down to the problem of searching after your knees, if there may be a few trouble, what's interesting is how awesome people view the hassle, and greater to the factor, the answer.

Have you ever heard of the tale approximately the 5 men telling each one-of-a-type what they have been preserving onto?

As said in Wikipedia:

"A organization of blind guys heard that a weird animal, referred to as an elephant, had been delivered to the metropolis, but none of them had been aware about its form and form. Out of curiosity, they stated: "We want to test out and recognize it by way of manner of way of touch, of which we are succesful". So, they sought it out, and when they located it they groped approximately it. In the case of the number one individual, whose hand landed on the trunk, stated "This being is sort of a thick snake".

"For each other one whose hand reached its ear, it regarded like a form of fan. As for each different man or woman, whose hand end up upon its leg, stated, the elephant is a pillar like a tree-trunk. The blind guy who positioned his hand upon its aspect said, "elephant is a wall". Another who felt its tail, defined it as a rope. The final felt its tusk, maintaining the elephant is that that is tough, smooth and prefer a spear."

People have a tendency to recognise to ideas of what some thing is, and often, they base their solution on their confined idea. In this specific case, the 'elephant' is "the treatment for knee issues".

In 1982 an MIT professor attributed an example of the saying to [the famous psychologist] Maslow as advised inside the "New York Times": thirteen

"Abraham Maslow as quickly as said that to him who has quality a hammer, the whole international looks as if a nail," stated Joseph Weizenbaum, a professor of laptop technology at M.I.T.

So what does this need to do with knee pain

and looking after your knees?

The reality is that looking after your knees can help lessen knee pain. Knees are pretty complex, with splendid types of tissues, at the side of bones, cartilage, tendons, and ligaments. Things can cross wrong with any of them. That moreover method that there are numerous strategies to cope with knee issues.

But the difficulty is, many specialists or groups have one product to promote, which they'll nicely portray as "The Magic Bullet". Surgeons regularly see surgical remedy as the solution to knee problems, and but, studies additionally display that going to two one-of-a-type physicians will yield unique diagnoses, not to mention remedies or solutions.

Lack of Objective Advice

Depending on who you communicate to, you could well get without a doubt specific advice. Here is my personal lifestyles revel in for example.

The first time I tore my knee cartilage, I became sitting on a bus, the bus lurched, I felt a twinge in my knee, and shortly, I have become hobbling spherical, and my knee have become swollen. At the time, in 1984, the most effective answer I knew of have become surgical procedure, so the clinical medical doctor removed a quarter of my meniscus.

Thirty years later, I became sitting skip-legged and felt a twinge in my knee, which I possibly angry by means of the use of going to a too strenuous yoga elegance in step with week later. I even have grow to be despite the fact that on foot spherical, but the ache end up terrible. An MRI determined that the meniscus had fractured further, and that the cartilage in my knee became frayed. That's truely what it felt like, sort of like gravel or sandpaper in my knee joint, not the brilliant clean feeling we want to have.

So I have been given surgical procedure a 2d time. The doc stated, "This will very last about five years, you received't need a knee possibility now". Which appeared like a prediction that I didn't need fulfilled. Let's face it. Surgery sucks.

Two years later, I modified into doing correct enough, the usage of my bicycle round town, it's miles both fun and great workout for the knee joint.

Unless a few silly bike motive force rides proper into your knee, that is what came about.

They took me to the hospital, X-ray confirmed no damaged bones however I couldn't walk for 3 weeks, nor placed any weight on it. An orthopedist did a check and said he notion it have grow to be a pulled ACL, the indoors ligament in the knee. Fortunately although, now not torn, which would possibly have proven a number of swelling. Not to say want for reconstructive surgical remedy.

He advocated a few medication that sounded adore it had more element consequences than I need to hazard.

What to do? I went to every other medical doctor, and recommended him

I preferred to appearance the physical therapist accessible at the sanatorium.

Get a Second Medical Opinion

and Trust Your Judgment

She gave a totally amazing prognosis than the primary doctor. Basically, a muscle and ligament pressure but now not so excessive. She proceeded to address me in now not one or , but 4 one-of-a-kind strategies! Moist heat, cold, Ultrasound, and TENS, or Transcutaneous Electrical Nerve Stimulation.

The physical therapist furthermore gave me a few specific bodily bodily video games that I may additionally moreover need to do.

The remedies truely helped, however additionally opened my eyes to the truth that, to combine metaphors about elephants and hammers, 'There is multiple manner to pores and pores and pores and skin a cat'.

So, here's a listing of different approaches of treating sore knees yourself:

1.   Rest

2.   Ice

three.   Compression

four.   Elevation

five.   NSAID medicine, prescription or non prescription

6.   Herbal remedies (e.G. Turmeric, Ginger, Pepper)

7.   Exercise/self bodily remedy

Yoga

weight education with machines

weight education with out machines

eight.   Get the right form of shoes

9.   Maintain healthy weight

10.Knee braces

magnetic tourmaline, copper, bamboo, and so on.

11.Compression Knee sleeves (severa kinds as in knee braces)

12.Knee straps

13.Velcro secured knee wraps

14.Gel knee braces

15.Knee pads

sixteen.Joint supplement tablets/drugs

vitamins, minerals, herbs

17.Pain treatment machines

Cold laser

heat,

infrared warm temperature pad and pen,

infrared heat lamp

ultrasound remedy

TENS, EMS, ICT, PENS

18.Self Massage

19.Topical Ointments and salves

Tiger Balm

Bengay

magnesium oil

20.Analgesic sprays, patches

21.Foods–proper weight loss plan options

suitable sufficient fiber

anti inflammatory food, end result vegetables

keep away from sugary, processed junk food, alcohol

22.Superfoods

23.Magnetic treatment

24.Acupressure, self implemented

25.Stop smoking

26. Reduce day by day lifestyles strain through rest, meditation

Making Sense of Your Choices

Nowadays, we get hundreds of advertisements of a wide variety. However, an entire lot of the time, we don't understand in which to look. The motive of this report is to SAVE YOU TIME. Based by myself experience as a knee ache victim, I did many loads of hours of research over numerous years and got here up with a listing of things you yourself can do to deal with your knees. As the listing above indicates, you have got pretty some choices!

My motive isn't to diagnose. That is the role for a clinical expert. But the reality is that there is a lot you may do to assist yourself, if you have suitable records. Not each this type of remedies will provide you with the outcomes you want, and that is without a doubt now not what I advocate. What this does do, is offer you with a few resources to check for your private.

So, permit's dive in to this listing of things you could do.

R.I.C.E.

We aren't speaking approximately making sushi proper right here. These are the maximum number one subjects you could do even as you experience discomfort or swelling.

It may also moreover appear apparent, but quite some us diehard athletes count on we're able to push through the ache. Trust your body! You are feeling ache, ache, aching, and so on for a purpose. There is a time to be a hero and a time to behave appropriately. Know at the same time as to prevent and take a relaxation, both in a exercising, going for walks, or other hobby. Or an prolonged period. Even severa days or every week if vital. If the hassle however hasn't lengthy past away, you probably have to are trying to find professional help.

Soreness, pain and discomfort is regularly the end result of infection. The body tissues are reacting to a stressor. Applying ice can lessen irritation given that it's miles Cold, obviously. You can use ice in a plastic bag, wrapped in cloth. Or you may get gel wraps that you preserve in the freezer.

Compress the Knee Using a Bandage or Sleeve. Doing so will help restrict the amount of swelling caused to the knee. You can either use a bandage or sleeve to compress the knee. These are usually presented on-line and at drug stores. The compression may additionally moreover assist with useful resource and every so often allows with knee ache and stiffness.

Elevation can relieve swelling, and permit fluids to drain out of the vicinity, that might then assist with drift

Chapter 5: Prescription Or Non-Prescription

If you make a decision to transport the route of taking medicinal drug, the first question to ask yourself is Prescription in preference to OTC (OTC stands for Over the Counter. These are drugs which might be quite honestly available without seeing a doctor first). The trouble of selection is not surely due to the hassle in evaluating treatment functions.

Aside from the prescribed medication for joint ache, there also are powerful over the counter painkillers that make the selection way quite difficult. Thus, prescription in vicinity of OTC is the problem. Read the labels cautiously; observe the experts and cons, to make a clever desire. Consider your contemporary-day health situation and desires. Determine whether or not or now not the medication can deal with your troubles or not especially when you have hypersensitive reactions. In addition, offer hobby to the aspect consequences and reactions.

The unique component is truely consolation and fee. Heading all the way proper all the way down to your close by Walgreen's, CVS, or nearby drug maintain or chemist's preserve (if you live within the UK) is a lot faster than searching forward to a doctor's appointment, which can also nicely entail the physician's charge, then getting a prescription which can also fee masses more and take extra time, than just grabbing some aspirin or Tylenol off the shelf.

Prescription Medication to Treat Your Knee Pain

Doctors typically prescribe prescription remedy, inside the case of a extra extreme scenario, collectively with rheumatoid arthritis. Rheumatoid arthritis is due to an autoimmune scenario, which leads to irritation, pain and redness.

One of the most common prescribed drugs for knee pain is the disorder-enhancing anti-rheumatic capsules or DMARDS. These capsules decrease contamination, ease ache and decrease signs and symptoms and symptoms and signs and symptoms. Common DMARDs are Trexall, Plaquenil, and Azulfidine.

Prescribed biologics are often used with DMARDs whilst the latter do no longer paintings properly for knee pain. The prescribed remedy is injectable. It reduces contamination in sufferers, except for humans with contamination or sensitive immunity. Common examples of biologics are Rituxan, Remicade, Orencia and Actemra. Be certain to thoroughly understand those in advance than signing as lots as take them, regardless of the fact that.

If DMARDs and biologics do no longer offer you with the consequences you want, medical doctors may additionally prescribe Janus associated kinase inhibitors. The inhibitors art work via affecting the immune cell hobby and genes. Joint and tissue harm is probably halted with the resource of these capsules. They moreover assist in avoiding infection. Examples of the inhibitors are baricitinib and tofacitinib.

Over-the-Counter Medicines for Arthritis Relief

Over-the-counter medicine for knee ache is available in splendid bureaucracy and types. One of the usually used OTC drug remedies for joint pain is Tylenol moreover called Acetaminophen. The remedy can deal with mild to mild knee and hip pain.

However, patients with excessive blood strain, coronary coronary heart sickness and diabetes or other clinical circumstance truly have to speak over with their physician to keep away from detrimental drug interactions or viable side results.

Non-steroidal anti-inflammatory capsules or NSAIDs are most well-known in treating arthritis pain. Most not unusual examples are aspirin, naproxen and Motrin. They sell dual motion treatment inside the direction of joint swelling and ache comfort. However, please be aware that every so often they have dangerous issue consequences.

Pain relieving rubs are options for folks who do no longer need to take capsules or pills. They numb the pain by using manner of visiting through your pores and pores and skin. However, it want to not be considering oral ache relievers. The question of Prescription versus OTC arises regardless of drug treatments for outside use.

The Choice of Knee Pain Treatment

Largely Depends on You

The specialists and cons of prescription instead of OTC tablets take some cautious consideration. There are cons within the use of pharmaceuticals because of a few drug reactions. On the other hand, OTC capsules can also additionally have their cons in phrases of health risks. To make the proper choice on your knee ache treatment, remember your modern-day state of affairs. Do you've got got hypersensitive reactions or current health issues? Before you use any prescription or OTC drug, make sure it's going to no longer get worse the symptoms and signs and symptoms.

Moreover, in advance than selecting prescription rather than OTC capsules, take into account the severity of your ache. OTC tablets are frequently allowable in treating mild pain. If you without a doubt find it hard to choose, you can are searching for recommendation out of your clinical medical doctor. A professional knows the maximum suitable knee trouble drug if you need to avoid thing results. Alternatively, you can select a more herbal knee safety, along with Ayurvedic remedies, or extraordinary natural or domestic treatments.

Herbal Remedies

There are traditional medicinal practices used each within the West and within the East, on the side of Naturopathy and Homeopathy in the West, and in the East, Indian Ayurvedic remedy, or Chinese Traditional Medicine. These constitute up to 5000 years of information handed down through the a long time. In reality, many contemporary-day drug remedies are derived from vegetation.

The massive drug agencies tweak them, patent them and then sell for a large earnings, while herbal treatments may go actually as properly. Examples are Turmeric, Pepper, Ginger, in reality to call 3. Obviously, a whole list and talk is past the scope of this document. But the factor is, that there are some of options besides the pricey and in all likelihood risky prescription drug direction.

Exercise and Self Physical Therapy

Some people want to exercise at home, each with weights or device, at the same time as others like getting out of the house and going to the gym. There are masses of techniques to workout. Here are a few examples.

Yoga

Yoga has been used for masses of years for developing calmness, flexibility and awareness. It can assist loosen up and manual muscle groups and boom circulate to joints. There are many yoga publications every on-line and in instructions.

Physical Therapy Exercises

If you have were given had been given joint and particularly knee problems, a physical therapist can be able to assist. While they have got splendid varieties of machines and other place of business treatments, an splendid physical therapist can advise the proper sorts of carrying events which will help and assist heal your knee, at the identical time as heading off wearing activities or behaviors which irritate it.

Weight Training Exercise at the Gym

If you have got a few enjoy running out with weights. You can exercise on your very very own. Even despite the fact that strolling out with a partner will permit you to live steady, and inspire each one-of-a-kind. On the opportunity hand, when you have not worked out with weights, and especially so with fitness center weight machines, it's an extremely good concept to get familiar with people with the assist of a private teacher. Most gyms have human beings in particular skilled to assist.

Exercise Machines, which encompass Ellipticals, Stationary Cycles and Rowing Machines.

Going to a health club is a brilliant manner to construct average body electricity. Gyms have unique machines to focus on specific regions, collectively together together with your knees. Rowing machines have 8 benefits, for instance. Plus, they work 5 muscle businesses.

You can also use the services of a non-public trainer, who may also advise things you can do to help your knees. Please observe, even though, that while you exercise consultation with weights, there's a higher risk of harm. So be cautious.

Home sporting events with minimum tool

If you don't want to pay for a gymnasium, you could do many knee strengthening physical video games, which embody yoga and electricity constructing sports activities using smooth weights or perhaps simply your personal frame weight and some homemade gadgets. For example, doing leg will increase with a bucket on your ankle offers weight even using a wall to do sure varieties of carrying occasions can artwork. There are many domestic bodily video video games you may try in case you do some research.

Get the Right Kind of Shoes

The problem with knees is that if the meniscus and cartilage, the natural marvel absorbers, can put on out, meaning there may be not anything to take inside the shock of thigh and decrease leg bones hitting each exceptional, inflicting ache. That's why getting footwear with precise surprise absorbency can assist compensate. Shoes with leather-based soles typically don't have that, however there are accurate comfortable footwear, or maybe orthopedic footwear specially designed to beneficial resource your knees.

Chapter 6: Maintain Healthy Weight

Did you recognize that each pound of greater weight you've got is identical to 4 pounds for your knees! That's due to the truth the burden of your body is focused on the smaller region of your knee joint, unlike joints on your better body. Weight has turn out to be a huge trouble these days.

We are continuously bombarded with advertisements telling us to devour junk food, rapid food, chemically loaded food, with hundreds of synthetic elements, and too many carbohydrates, whilst we should be consuming more quit give up result, greens and protein.

If you are considerably obese, lay off the ones high-quality massive bowls of spaghetti, mashed potatoes, pizza, cookies, and in particular the packaged substances like potato and corn chips. Drastically reduce the starch and boom greens to ease starvation.

Stop the fizzy sugary liquids, the white bread, cakes, cookies, and tremendous fatty elements like bacon and hamburgers fried in grease.

Knee Braces, Sleeves, Wraps and Straps

There are a great style of what's substantially known as Orthotics. That is, external appliances to wear on the knee. We'll deliver a quick assessment of what those are, even though an extensive clarification goes beyond the record.

Knee braces with 'Sticky' straps

These famous knee home equipment are worn through using the use of covering the knee joint and the usage of hook and loop fastener straps to constant it. You can modify the tightness to a point and they will be adjustable for precise length knees. They may also have accessories, collectively with magnets, or occasionally tourmaline that's been activated to mirror once more your frame's natural warmth. For the three exceptional knee manual braces, study this file.

Knee Compression Sleeves

These are tubular—you pull them on over your foot and slide them up over the knee. They are regularly made from specific forms of materials and function specialised capabilities. Some examples consist of magnetic compression knee sleeves, which include magnets, reputed to have healing houses.

Some sleeves are made from neoprene, an synthetic rubber, which naturally compresses the joint. Others use latex elastic, together with cotton, for a easy herbal feeling the neoprene fashion, despite the fact this is likewise pretty snug.

Variations encompass copper infused cloth, for the motive that some people revel in that copper (because of its excessive electric powered powered conductivity) embedded fabric improves float as well as prevents infection. Bamboo based fabric is likewise said to have soothing homes and these days, bamboo is made into very snug fiber.

Knee Straps

These are a smaller version of the sleeves and braces. Basically, about an inch-big strap that suits throughout the knee beneath the joint. These are useful for runners or in case you need to alleviate tendon troubles.

Knee Wraps

Long strips of cloth which bind the knee with the useful resource of way of wrapping across the joint. They are a number of the oldest knee gadgets for each protective the knee within the direction of sports, and soothing the joint that has the extra hassle of feeling volatile.

Gel Knee Braces

This as a substitute new kind brace consists of gel, to behave as a shock absorber, similarly to relying on the gel, much like the concept referred to earlier, using cold to help with the infection.

Knee Pad

These are worn throughout sports, due to the fact they guard the knee from falls or in case you are doing artwork for your knees, like putting tiles on a floor. That difficult ground can get effective painful, and knee pads can assist.

For a greater certain communicate of 12 Different Kinds of Knee Supports for one in all a kind functions, go HERE.

Joint Supplements: Vitamins, Minerals,

Herbs, Nature Based Chemicals

There are innumerable products for alleviating joint ache, or knee ache.

Here is a brief list. The number one topics I search for are the sort of components, the quantity of additives in a dose, and cost. The fact is that there are some of right products, but, there is no person product that has 'all' the fine materials. To buy they all is probably loopy high priced, and besides, who wants to consume bowls entire of drugs and capsules?

Here is a partial list of substances to search for in supplements:

Vitamins: Vitamin C, Vitamin D

Minerals: boron, magnesium, manganese, chromium, copper, zinc

Herbal/plant based really: Boswellia, Curcumin from Turmeric, Ginger, Piperine from Black Pepper, astaxanthin, pycnogenol, grape seed extract

Natural chemical substances produced via the body: MSM, Hyaluronic Acid, Cetyl Myristoleate (derived from herbal frame chemical,) Glucosamine, Chondroitin

One brand I like and use is Joint Regen. It has 12 precise elements as shown on this infographic.

Pain Treatment Machines

Recently, increasingly more options to the drug or surgical remedy route have turn out to be available. Some have greater sorting out at the back of them than others, however, many humans have become unique outcomes with various ache remedy machines that use energy.

Cold laser, (additionally known as low-degree laser treatment or LLLT)

Heating pad

Infrared warmth pad

Infrared Lamp

Laser pen

ultrasound remedy

TENS (Transcutaneous Electrical Nerve Stimulation

EMS (Electrical Muscle Stimulation)

ICT (Interferential Current Therapy)

PENS (Percutaneous Electrical Nerve Stimulation

Topical Ointments, Patches and Sprays

Rather than swallowing tablets that could have an effect in your entire body, while what you really want is right now treatment on the particular joint, there are pretty a few options of topical products. Some are extra orientated inside the direction of Western medicinal drug, including Bengay or Aspercreme, on the same time as others are like Chinese medication, the very well-known Tiger Balm, which has comparable factors as Bengay plus a few others.

There are sprays you can attempt, together with Biofreeze, which acts similarly to icing the joint. Aspercreme has a compound with Salicylate, that is related to Aspirin. There is likewise a product with Lidocaine, a community anaesthetic.

In addition, you may use patches. Patches have the gain of going right now on the affected location, and there is no wastage, that you get at the equal time as you spray. Likewise, the patches have the medication without delay in contact together together with your pores and pores and skin, which absorbs it.

If you use lotions or ointments, some of it might rub off in your clothes, so you lose some and every now and then they may go away a stain at the garments. So you've got a choice of sprays, ointments or patches for immediate topical consolation proper on the affected joint.

Chapter 7: Proper Diet Choices

One of the biggest stressful situations we are going through in recent times is food and diet. We are affected in the following strategies:

Long Distance between Farm and Table Nowadays, meals is grown a long way from in which we absolutely devour it. Studies have tested that the not unusual distance a few of the farm and the table within the USA is 1000 miles. The meals are mostly a week antique earlier than we even purchase it! So a great deal of the freshness and strength of the meals is out of place

Widespread use of chemical fertilizers and pesticides This moreover effects inside the loss of micronutrients that might usually be determined in meals this is grown in the 'virtuous circle' of herbal agriculture. When animals and flowers have interaction with every specific, they nourish each other. When meals is grown the usage of chemical substances, vitamins is misplaced. What's worse, the meals may also have pollution from the chemical substances themselves.

GMO's or Genetically Modified Organisms, this is, ingredients which have their genetic shape messed with inside the intervening time are being identified as a supply of plenty of fitness issues, from allergic reactions to infertility. Because they exist outside of actual nature, they act as stressors on our our our bodies, which may be pressured out sufficient as it is.

Use of peculiar components, together with food coloring, flavor enhancers, stabilizers and so on. The pleasant thing we're capable of do to avoid those is to avoid packaged and processed foods when possible. Always observe labels for additives. If you spot a few ordinary terms, which means it's miles a few chemical additive that we humans aren't designed to consume. So don't devour them, if possible!

Too heaps sugar. Sugar intake is through the roof. Our our our bodies can not cope with the amount of sugar in foods. That motives rapid burning and generally infection. Not to say weight problems and ultimately, diabetes in which your pancreas truely cannot way the sugar any more.

Too an awful lot alcohol. Alcohol is a short burning fuel for the frame, and subsequently ends up being stored as fats, and stresses out special organs. In unique, eating beer can increase the risk of gout, a completely painful joint disease, with the resource of two hundred% in folks that drink beers an afternoon, vs. Non drinkers.

Too masses food, in stylish. Fact is, weight problems, or being drastically overweight, locations extremely good pressure at the joints in addition to considered one of a kind organs.

Improve Your Food Habits with the ones guidelines

Eat masses greater quit result and veggies. Organic if the least bit feasible

Try to eat locally grown elements sold at your neighborhood farmers' marketplace

Avoid GMO - genetic animal materials. That is hard to do nowadays, but it's miles possible. Farmed Salmon, as an instance.

Read labels. If it looks like a weird chemical, assume   times in advance than shopping for and ingesting.

Eat less sugar, within the shape of desserts, cookies, sweet, clean liquids

Drink lots less alcohol

Eat fairly. Try fasting for at the least one half of day every week, to offer your digestive device a relaxation. Plus, whilst you speedy on a regular foundation, your body learns to burn off fats.

Consider intermittent fasting, this means that that that no longer consuming for 12-18 hours all through a 24 hour cycle

Superfoods

There has been masses of discussion about Superfoods, which p.C. Greater nutrients in them than regular substances. They can also have greater protein than their everyday counterparts, an instance being Quinoa in location of Rice.

They may additionally additionally have big amounts of Vitamin C or distinctive nutrients, which incorporates rose hips in place of oranges.

Specialty fish oil has immoderate nutritive content material, and can useful useful resource in healing joints in contrast with greater not unusual oils like corn or soy oils. Fish oil is not a few trouble you'd use for cooking however alternatively, taken as a complement.

One possible downside to superfoods is that they may be not as successfully available as ordinary factors, and similarly they may be pretty lots extra steeply-priced. Advocates say the price is properly well worth it. For example, wheat grass juice crafted from freshly grown wheat that has surely sprouted and is in its early grassy degree earlier than developing the actual wheat grains, may be very expensive, and has for use glowing.

You can get wheat grass extract that has been dried, so the growing and processing adds to the fee. This is virtually one example. On the alternative hand, there may be a few evidence that those meals are so powerful that they are able to save you or even treatment disorder. For your loose report on Superfoods, flow HERE.

Stop Smoking

This recommendation to prevent smoking has been remarkable for severa many years, ever because the tobacco enterprise come to be in the long run known as to account for the reality that smoking is unstable in plenty of processes. If you smoke, you're growing your opportunities of multiple health problems, no longer actually knee or joint ache. So do remedy to prevent smoking.

Reduce Stress and Pay Attention

to Your Emotional Health

One of the splendid advances within the past forty or so years is the belief that our our our bodies and minds are plenty more integrated than have grow to be formerly belief. If you revel in strain in a unmarried area of your life, you can well enjoy signs and signs and signs in exclusive regions of your lifestyles. Looking at your complete wonderful of existence is a sensible method. Learn relaxation or respiratory and meditation strategies to govern pain.

Complementary and Alternative

Medical Therapies

This very last segment deals with methods to cope with ache which is probably perhaps a long way afield or in a few states, even unlawful. Medical marijuana is one example. Here is a listing of a few strategies to keep in mind.

Magnetic Therapy makes use of magnets to lessen ache. There is full-size controversy over whether or not this sort of treatment is natural hype, or simply has a systematic foundation.

Medical Marijuana. Many human beings insist that numerous additives of the marijuana plant which include cannabinols can prompt relaxation and ache comfort. However, in masses of jurisdictions, it's far taken into consideration as unstable as opioids and is exactly illegal

Reiki. This shape of remedy includes the conscious use of 'recovery energy' by means of a professional practitioner, to help heal the frame. You can use reiki for self remedy if you recognize what you are doing.

www.ingramcontent.com/pod-product-compliance
Lightning Source LLC
Chambersburg PA
CBHW071235020426
42333CB00015B/1481